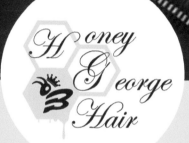

MENTAL AND SPIRITUAL WELLNESS

FOR THE POST-COVID-19 COSMETOLOGIST

ROBIN "HONEY" GEORGE

ISBN 978-1-63844-790-0 (paperback)
ISBN 978-1-63844-791-7 (digital)

Christian Faith Publishing, Inc.
832 Park Avenue
Meadville, PA 16335
www.christianfaithpublishing.com

Limitation of liability/disclaimer of warranty: while the publisher and author have used their best efforts in preparing this guide and workbook, they make no representations or warranties with respect to the accuracy or completeness of the contents of this document and specifically disclaim any implied warranties of merchantability or fitness for particular purpose. No warranty may be created or extended by sales representatives, promoters, or written sales materials.

The advice and strategies contained herein may not be suitable for your situation. You should consult with a professional where appropriate. Neither the publisher nor author shall be liable for any loss of profit or any other commercial damages, including but not limited to special, incidental, consequential, or other damages. Due to the dynamic nature of the internet, certain links and website information contained in this publication may have changed. The author and publisher make no representations to the current accuracy of the web information shared.

Printed in the United States of America

TABLE OF CONTENTS

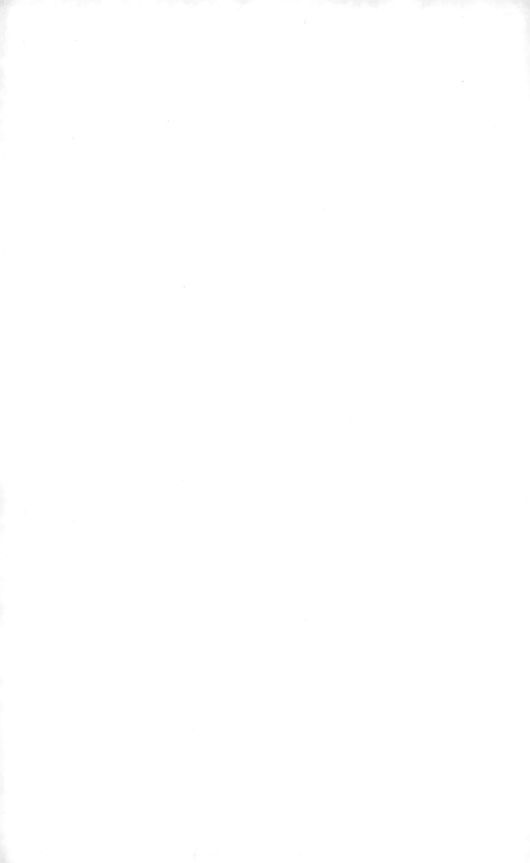

INTRODUCTION

In March of 2020, the government called for our nation to go into a complete lockdown. Any service that was considered nonessential was put on pause with no replay in sight. It was a devastating time across all of the socioeconomic statuses.

Everything was uncertain. Even the small things that we could always count on were no longer guaranteed. Parents had to become in-home teachers. Toilet paper was out of stock everywhere. People resorted to making homemade hand sanitizer. The movie theaters shut down. The playgrounds shut down. Churches shut down. Grocery items were limited. And of course, the salon industry came to a screeching halt!

While some corporate employees could switch gears and just work from home, the independent contractors, on the other hand, had no initial support. The state-funded unemployment benefits did not recognize the salon industry as recipients of such aid.

In my failed attempts to process the new normal, God afforded me some dynamic opportunities to build faith as well as my hope in Him! In my studying about faith and revelation knowledge fostered by Him, I now look at the particular set of circumstances surrounding the beauty professional experience, and I feel capable to assist.

This book was birthed from the countless days of learning to adjust expectations, resetting some counterproductive mental processes, and most importantly connecting to God!

Section 1.

MENTAL WELLNESS

Think about What You're Thinking

Imagine your alarm goes off in the morning, you open your eyes, and a flood of thoughts, responsibilities, and emotions start to race in your mind. The struggle for the balance between work and home begins to compete. It's said that the average human being makes thirty-five thousand microdecisions in the course of a single day. Things like what to wear, breakfast options, punctuality, getting kids off to school, the work commute, returning text messages, scheduling date night, booking clients, remembering your face masks, zoom calls, coworker relations, product inventory, guilt from past failures, pressure to perform services well, social media posting, shortcomings, insecurities, the bad client review, etc.

(Your list may look something like this or not, but the point is that upon waking up in the morning, sometimes there is a barrage of thoughts regarding planning, stress, and worries that descends upon your conscious.)

So after spending the better part of the morning, stewing in the overwhelming thoughts and beginning to carry out today's responsibilities, you now start to experience the emotion of those thoughts. The nature of the thoughts that are put into rotation will determine the type of emotions that you take on.

For instance, if you let yesterday's salon altercation with your suitemate be the forefront of today's thoughts, then feelings of anger or resentment will most

MENTAL WELLNESS

likely be the result. Now you're faced with negatively charged feelings, a.k.a. a *bad mood*, and have moved on to acting in concordance. You walk into the work environment already on edge and subconsciously waiting for the other shoe to drop. With the salon environment being populated with all different kinds of personalities and potential triggers, it doesn't take long for the negative actions to rear its head.

Now imagine the next day. You just wake up and find yourself in a seemingly good mood without a cause. You just get up in the morning feeling good by default. It seems like things are going in your favor. You get a notification from Instagram because your work has been shared by a popular page, you look at your schedule, and you've got all confirmed clients paying high-end service prices. You get in your car, and your spouse has filled your tank.

You order your favorite morning coffee at Starbucks, and the car before you has already paid your order. You arrive at the salon and find money you

didn't know you misplaced in your work apron. You get great tips all day. All your clients are loving their results today. And to top it all off, the bulk of your favorite musician's songs have made their way to the Pandora or Apple music playlist. (I've always enjoyed good music to work to.)

You have good interactions with clients and coworkers. Even a few remarks about what a good day you must be having because of the way you are floating around the salon.

Although these are two seemingly different workday experiences, the bottom line is still the same. In both cases, the direction of how the day went was not controlled by the stylist but by the reaction to circumstances. In the case of the bad day, there was a wave of stressors that started in the mind and went unchecked. Those thoughts turned into emotions, and then the stylist began to act out what first started in the mind. In the case of the good day, the stylist woke up having good feelings and then went on to experience good fortune throughout the day, all of which yielded good actions by the individual. Don't get me wrong; having a great day is always the goal. However, the stylist never purposed to be happy.

It just happened. This trains our minds to think that we have to feel like whatever we are experiencing, and feelings are sometimes liars! We can't rely on them.

What I'm saying is that there is a danger to walking around with thoughts that are there by default. Essentially, we are turning over the influence of our very minds to external factors. At this rate, we won't experience a good day until it's *handed* to us by things lining up. On the other hand, our good day can be ruined by things lining up to oppose us.

Don't get me wrong; I used to do life being unintentional in my thoughts and emotions. However, the season of COVID-19 helped me realize that I have to be purposeful about approaching each day and every day. The moment I let up, the outside influence is

ready to engage and allow the external to influence the internal. I challenge you to begin to speak to your day as well. Our words have power. And believe me, one day we shall reap what we say.

As independent contractors, it's often like being a one-man band. There are a lot of pressures that come with the business. These pressures are present each and every workday. The stylist must keep an efficient time schedule behind the chair.

There is an expectation of executing a hair service as perfectly as the clients see on Pinterest, Facebook, and YouTube. We hold ourselves accountable to stay current with our services, which means spending time and money on continuing education classes.

Post-COVID, we now have more expectations to uphold a more intensive standard of sanitation in keeping the public safe. The new Instagram algorithm requires that we change the way we market and convert to sales. This new education of learning Internet marketing requires time and money to learn the new system and be successful. As we rebuild our businesses from the ground up, that means learning or hiring help for proper accounting of what we spend and earn.

That's just the tip of the iceberg! Externally, there are websites and apps dedicated to offering people more avenues to rate us, validate us, popularize us, blacklist us, and "whatever else us" that one off-day behind the chair can cause. So you can see how important it is for one to have mental wellness, not only for the sake of ourselves but also for those we encounter. If we continue to entertain negative thought processes, then we just run around retriggering ourselves and/or one another repetitively.

I'll bet by now you're wondering, *What exactly is mental wellness? And how can I get some?* I'm glad you asked those questions. While there are different schools of thought that compete for the exact definition, I like to use this one. *Mental wellness* can be loosely defined as the ability to think, feel, and act in ways that create a positive impact on your physical and social well-being.

Notice it does not include the term *happiness*. Being mentally sound doesn't mean just acting happy all the time. It means thinking, feeling, and acting in ways that positively impact your total well-being.

Psychology most definitely supports that there is a correlation between what we're thinking, how we're feeling, and how we're acting. The theory is referred to as the cognitive behavior triangle (Aaron Beck 1960s). If we can change the way we think about negative things and even problematic people, it is safe to say that we can change our actions.

You ever wonder why the same negative event could happen to different people, but the responses all be different? Let's say you work hard at completing a hairstyle or haircut, and the first thing the guest says is a complaint about an area she finds unsatisfactory.

SECTION 1.

MENTAL WELLNESS

Why would one stylist take offense versus another stylist being happy to oblige?

It's because of what we say to ourselves when someone tells us that we "missed the mark."

You can think the complaint is an honest assessment, as a personal attack, or anything else in between. No matter which one you tell yourself, your actions will surely follow.

So what should we be telling ourselves in the face of a situation like this? Although most of us find our identity in what we do for a living, it is not. We have to remember to separate who we are from what we do.

Offense happens when something or someone relays contradiction to our belief of self. In essence, when we hear the complaint, we tell ourselves we are not good enough, and that hurts. So instead of thinking, *She complained about me*, think that, *She complained about it.*

It is separate from *me* and therefore is a safe and more accurate way to view the claim. Now, I don't have to own this burden of judgment and can feel different emotions that will allow me to act accordingly.

I offer another sample scenario where criticism can either hurt or offend. Negative customer feedback is just a part of business. We dealt with the "unhappy about a service" customer scenario, so now let's tackle a "rude about the service" customer. In this scenario, you service a client and honestly do your best to oblige what was discussed in the consultation. The client looks at the finished product and responds far differently than the client who simply complained. What if this client caused a scene, yelled, personally insulted you, and used *choice* words in conversation with you? It's a lot harder to employ the separate *you* from *it* because of the aggressive attack on you. The first thing you should understand is the *anatomy* of a rude person. When people are rude by default, they lack the tools to process their emotions. Usually, the triggering moment is not about the moment at all. It's not about you. You have to employ a little empathy to deal

MENTAL WELLNESS

with this type of person because they are handling a multitude of overwhelming situations. Can you imagine the kinds of inner turmoil that must be going on inside the mind of a person in order to muster up that type of aggravated response to someone servicing them? Remember: Think. Feel. Act. Imagine a house being on fire.

Would it deescalate the situation by lighting more fire to the existing fire? No, right? Firemen show up to put out the fire with water. That's exactly the role we need to take on in dealing with rude people. Be the water and not the fire. I realize what I'm saying is very counterculture. The social norm is to fight fire with fire. But this is business. As professionals, we seek to serve and earn, not tear down and win fights.

I would like to challenge you to think about what you're thinking. Use my mental checklist to evaluate what you say to yourself with and without conflict. The object is to determine what you say to yourself on the regular.

MENTAL WELLNESS

Think about What I'm Thinking

Am I having anger thoughts?

Anger tells us that someone owes me something that I feel I deserve. What do you feel you are owed and why? Will your life change if you can't have it?

Yes ☐   No ☐

Am I having guilt thoughts?

Guilt tells us that we owe someone something that we cannot repay. What do you feel you owe and why? Will your life if you are not forgiven?

Yes ☐   No ☐

Am I having greed thoughts?

Greed tells us that we owe ourselves more than we need. Why do you want to have more? For you? For someone else?

Yes ☐   No ☐

Am I having jealous thoughts?

Jealousy tells us that someone owes us something we deserve over another person. Why do you feel that you deserve something that the other person does not? Will your life change if you do not get what you want?

Yes ☐   No ☐

Sidenote:

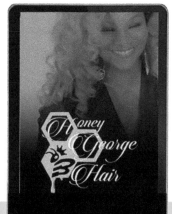

Oftentimes, when we examine the reasons behind our thoughts, we get to the real motive. Talking it out will sift out the validity of the things we think we have to have. It's important to ask yourself questions and give yourself honest answers. Are your reasons unselfish, reasonable, honest, and fair?

SECTION 1.

MENTAL WELLNESS

Am I having fear thoughts?   Yes   No

Fear tells us that there is danger. It can be rational and appropriate or irrational and inappropriate. Which are you dealing with? Why are you afraid?

Am I having anxiety thoughts?   Yes   No

Anxiety is referred to as the fight or flight trigger in the brain used to keep you safe from harm. Is the cause of your anxiety actually life-threatening? Why or why not?

Am I having worry thoughts?   Yes   No

Worry tells us the end result of our problem is uncertain or has the possibility of a negative result. Will the possible negative result be life-changing? How?

Am I having panic thoughts?   Yes   No

Panic is the sensation of fear. Is the cause of the panic rational or reflexive? Will it change your life in any significant way? How?

Hopefully, this exercise highlighted some misfires of thoughts and emotions. If a lot of these responses were yes, then I would urge you to seek a professional to talk with. (I've been to therapy myself.) There is no shame in seeking help.

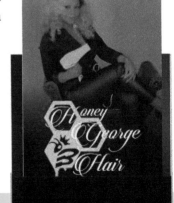

NOTES

_____

_____

_____

_____

_____

_____

_____

_____

_____

_____

_____

_____

_____

_____

_____

_____

_____

_____

_____

_____

_____

_____

_____

_____

_____

_____

_____

_____

NOTES

NOTES

_____
_____
_____
_____
_____
_____
_____
_____
_____
_____
_____
_____
_____
_____
_____
_____
_____
_____
_____
_____
_____
_____
_____
_____
_____

Section 2.

SPIRITUAL WELLNESS

Thought Content

I use caution with the following information because it is potentially dangerous knowledge for being set free from mental torment through the finished work of Jesus Christ!

Our thoughts originate from three sources of influence: humans or ourselves, God, or Satan.

You can almost instantly tell what thought you are entertaining based on the content. Human thoughts are characterized by logic, reasoning, and natural task-oriented subject matters. God-influenced thoughts tend to bear the fruits of His spirit (Galatians 5:22). With the small still voice, our thoughts tend to include love, joy, peace, patience, kindness, goodness, and faithfulness.

Satan-influenced thoughts, usually a loud inner voice, are characterized by thoughts of pride, selfishness, greed, lust, jealousy, envy, sloth, gluttony, evil-plotting and evil-planning, fear, and worry.

When I got this revelation about thought content, it immediately freed me from the guilt of the things that would seemingly zap into my mind. Have you ever been minding your own business, and a wicked thought just pop into your mind? I know I have, and it even happened during my prayer time! I used to think, *What a horrible person I must be to think that.* The truth of the matter is that I didn't think that—it was suggested to me, and because I owned the evil thought, I didn't

SPIRITUAL WELLNESS

check it. You have about thirty seconds to check the content of a thought and either keep or cancel it! God's Word says something about this. It asks us to bring into captivity every thought to the obedience of Christ (2 Corinthians 10:5). We now have the knowledge of the right and power to evict those Satan-induced thoughts from our minds.

What about a thought that comes against your confidence or your ability to produce? You can't do that! You will fail in front of everyone! What makes you think you deserve to be _____! No one will support you! You aren't talented enough! Keep entertaining these thoughts, and pair it with a scroll down of all the success stories on your Instagram. You will certainly find yourself feeling angry, jealous, and insignificant!

Recognize that those thoughts are not yours because you want to be successful. You paid to go to beauty school, you rented your workspace, you invested in your craft, you had a website built, and you are actively marketing to potential clients. You're walking the faith steps of someone who wants it!

God certainly approves your agenda to serve people via the talents He gave you. They're your gifts in the first place. So who does that leave dry, hating in the corner of your mind? That's right—Satan. Satan translates to "the accuser" in Hebrew, and that's mostly what he does.

The second part of winning this thought content battle is replacing the negative-planted suggestions with what the Word of God says about you.

So to those things Satan was trying to accuse me of believing, I would then apply that I can do all things through Christ who strengthens me (Philippians 4:13). "For I know the thoughts I think towards you, saith the Lord, thoughts of peace, and not of evil, to give you an expected end" (Jeremiah 29:11).

Greater is he that is in you, than he that is in the world (1 John 4:4).

To any thought that is trying to cause me to be afraid I say, God has not given a spirit of fear, but of love, and of power, and of a sound mind (2 Timothy 1:7).

MEDITATION

When I heard the word *meditate*, I pictured someone taking a certain yoga position in some sort of an external effort to clear their mind of all thoughts. Meditation is actually the opposite because it is an internal activity defined as the act of focusing one's thoughts. It means to ponder or to think on. So by that definition, anytime we channel our thoughts to hone in on a certain worry, agitation, fear, or unrighteous concept, then we are in mediation.

I know sometimes, when we have a lot on our plates as entrepreneurs, especially post-COVID, it is very easy to go into meditating about things going wrong. I am guilty of this myself. When I first started exercising control over my thoughts, I had to constantly remind myself of a couple of things.

Number 1, get it out of my head and on paper. I got this concept from God's word. Many secular planners use this method because it is an effective principle.

In the book of Habakkuk 2:2, God tells him to write the vision and make it plain upon tables. What this does is give your mind the break it needs from having to remember the fine details for execution, a.k.a. worrying.

Number 2 is faith and works. Once I have written the plan, then I begin to walk it out with faith in God and trust in the abilities He has given me. "For as the body without the spirit is dead, so faith without works is dead also" (James 2:26).

If I find myself unable to stay away from ruminating thoughts, then I refer to what God says about those of us who have trouble shutting our minds down. He gives us healthy suggestions for what to think of. It is found in Philippians 4:8.

Fix your thoughts on what is true, honorable, right, pure, lovely, and admiral. Think about

SPIRITUAL WELLNESS

things that are excellent and worthy of praise. Then it goes on into the promise attached to this practice. Verse 9 says keep putting into practice all you learned and received from me—everything you heard and saw me doing. Then the peace of God will be with you.

I'll bet you are thinking that this bubble gum, candy-coated biblical resolution stuff is not going to work in the face of a real problem. I understand that thought process because I used to think that as well. No offense, but that type of thinking is just the luxury of inexperience and probably a little bit of self-reliance. It takes a real step of faith to surrender yourself to the Lord. When faced with difficult situations, I used to meditate on my problem so much that to me, it became larger than my God! In my mind, it seemed like my problems in business and in life were either too small or too large for God to handle. I felt like my only option was to handle it all on my own.

I remember one time I had a client that came to get a $250 service from me. She left happy but later disputed my charge with her bank, stating that she hadn't gotten a service at all! I was livid because I had worked very hard on her hair, and to then have the full amount of the service be later removed from my bank balance was unfair for me. I remember thinking about it hard and telling every friend or family member who would listen to me rant about the audacity of the young lady. I did everything in my power to prove my case and get the funds recovered. However, the case dragged on for the better part of a week. I finally got so frustrated by the situation that I then decided to invite God into my circumstance and ask for His help. That didn't stop my mind from constantly attempting to reflect on what happened and that I still was not awarded my rightful wages. It took some time and practice, but I had to be persistent in keeping my mind and my confessions in check.

I don't have to tell you that it got resolved because you probably guessed that I won the case.

The message I'm trying to highlight is not the beginning or

the ending but what happens during. It's the period of time between the conflict and the resolution. I'm asking, what are we focusing our thoughts on in that period of time? Are we concentrating on the money missing? Are we focusing on being offended? Are we planning and plotting revenge?

I'm not saying the answer is to just think positive, and the thing you want to happen will manifest. If the goal is to not allow the negative thought to become a negative emotion, then what should we think of? We have to control our thoughts and bring them into submission to God's word while we are going through the hard thing.

We still do the natural work that is required as we are standing in faith for the desired outcome. It's one of those things that are easy to do and easy not to do.

CONFESSIONS

Now that we have discussed the origin of our thoughts and what we should be thinking of in the *during*, the next thing on the docket is our confessions. Confessions could be defined as the fessing up to something, but that is not the type of confessions I'm getting at. I want to take a closer look at what we are actually saying in the *during* process or the words you allow to come out of your mouth.

Here's a great example! It's a Friday morning, and you're traveling to the salon. As you merge onto the freeway, you notice that there is a huge slowdown caused by one of those manufactured homes being transported on the back of a truck. Both lanes are blocked and reduced to a speed limit of ten miles per hour. Thoughts of your morning being ruined by your late arrival begin to swim about in your head. You think about how your whole day of back-to-back appointments is no longer going to be perfectly staggered for your much-needed breaks. Soon after that, the words to support those thoughts just roll off your tongue. "I am going to be so late." "I'll never catch up from this." "My whole schedule is going to be shot." "There goes my lunch break."

SPIRITUAL WELLNESS

You just went from thinking it to feeling it and now saying it! What's next? You guessed it. The next thing is acting like it already happened.

The word says a lot about our confessions. Our words have the power to bless or rob a situation. Proverbs 18:21 says that death and life are in the power of the tongue, and they who love it shall eat the fruit thereof. Even in a situation as mundane as traffic, we can shoot ourselves in the foot by speaking the worse possible outcomes.

In all my years of servicing clients, I have had so many different types of work schedules in order to accommodate the needs of my family. After my oldest daughter left for the navy, my in-home babysitter was gone. I changed my schedule to allow myself to drop the baby off at daycare and the elementary-aged one at school in the morning and pick them both up after school in the afternoon. My husband worked crazy early hours until the evening, so I worked in the salon while they were away at school.

When I tell you I had some super close calls in those years, I could *not* run late at the salon. It was just not an option. I had to be there to get my kids at the appointed times. There were many days where the clients would arrive late, my color didn't process correctly, or some other variations of problem that threatened my ability to take care of everything in a timely manner. I can honestly say that keeping my thoughts, meditations, and confessions in line with my desired outcome kept me successful in every area. I would call my husband and tell him some miraculous stories about how time just seemed to stand still to allow me to catch up, or I would get through a service in half of the service time. One day, I even started late, serviced all my booked clients, and left for the day earlier than my stop time! I absolutely would not allow my mouth to say anything other than overcoming statements! "I will get through my schedule on time and in time." "According to Numbers 13:30, I am well able to overcome."

"May the words of my mouth and the meditation of my heart

be pleasing to you, O Lord, my rock and my redeemer" (Psalms 19:14). I love to use this verse as a spiritual gauge. I ask myself, *Would the way I'm thinking about this be pleasing to God? Would I be proud or ashamed to say this thought to Him?* If the answer is no, then it must go! Our God has all power and all knowledge, and He can do anything! He is waiting for us to put our faith in Him and not our limited abilities so that He can and will make our way. As long as we are giving a voice to our defeated thoughts and cursing ourselves, then we cancel out His blessing for our circumstances.

PRAYING

When I was a little girl, my grandmother used to take me with her to her home church called Afton Villa Baptist Church in Baines, Louisiana. Every Sunday, there was a time during the service where one of the deacons would be granted the mic. This brother would get down on one knee and lead the church in prayer to the tune of the traditional gospel organ. The prayer was so eloquently stated as to who God

is, the power He possesses, and the pure reverence of the people. It was so powerful and perfectly stated. It was so perfectly stated that I was intimidated by the gold standard of prayer I witnessed. Prayer looked more like a talent I did not have rather than a communication. I'm not placing the blame for my lack of praying on this single instance. However, it was one thing in addition to other areas of ignorance that led to my bad perspective about prayer.

So then what is *prayer*? The simple answer is that it is a verbal communication between you and God. The type of communication where each party makes room for talking and listening.

There are also types of prayer. Prayers of worship and praise acknowledge God for who He is and recognize all that He does. Prayers of intercession and petition communicate to God on behalf of someone else. Prayers of supplication are seeking God and humbly asking Him of something in the spiritual or natural. Prayers of thanksgiving are communicating pure gratitude for all He has done, is

SECTION 2.

SPIRITUAL WELLNESS

doing, and will do for us specifically. Prayers of spiritual warfare are using our prayer to take a stance against the battles within ourselves and outward forces and also include seeking God's protection.

I think that for the purposes of this book, prayers of supplication are a great starting point. The reason I say that is because if I understood this principle correctly, then my choices in life would have been vastly different.

As I stated before, my prayer life sucked because I was looking at prayer through the wrong lens. I thought that you had to have a *prayer talent* of sorts to approach God. I thought you had to be scripturally versed to approach God. Most importantly, I thought you had to be *worthy* of His time to approach God. I didn't pray because I am none of those! I was so convinced of this false worthiness narrative that I was paralyzed in my faith walk. When I learned the significance of taking on the wardrobe of Christ, then that put away all my insecurities about coming to God.

You see, when we accept Christ, God no longer sees the shortcomings. He views us a righteous. Without Christ, the default is being viewed by our merit. And how God views our worldly merit is found in Isaiah 64:6. When we display our righteous deeds, they are nothing but filthy rags. So my problem was that I accepted Christ but had not adopted worthiness. I still had the worldview of righteousness being by my own merit.

I also did not have a good understanding of the relationship aspect. God is a good god, and He is like a concerned father who is interested in a relationship with his children. And there is no good thing He will withhold from us. Jesus talks about His parental goodness in Matthew 7:11. So if sinful people know how to give good gifts to their children, how much more will your heavenly Father give good gifts to those who ask him?

Another aspect that was wrapped up in my unwillingness to pray was thinking that God didn't love me. I believe He exists, and

SECTION 2.

I believed He loves other people more than me. (I know it's sad, but I'm just being honest.) I would see great things happen for other people and wonder, why not me? All the while, I never took any sacrificial time to get in communication with God. I had not even made my request known to Him. Nor had I made any steps toward that goal. Come to think of it, I may not have even wanted that blessing until I saw someone else receive it!

Don't get me wrong; I've had some great achievements in life during this time. Looking back, that was still attributed to God's goodness because I didn't deserve that either. In Matthew 5:45, Jesus says that our father gives His sunlight to both the evil and the good.

There is so much evidence in the word about God's loving nature. We can start with the foundation of our faith—John 3:16, "For God so loved the world that He gave His only begotten son." Romans 5:8 says, "God shows his great love for us by sending Christ to die for our sins while we were *still* sinners." Also

Romans 8:38 says that nothing can ever separate us from God's love. Neither death nor life, neither angels nor demons, neither our fears for today nor our worries about tomorrow—not even the powers of hell can separate us from God's love.

Then I adopted my personal foundational text about God's love in 1 John 4:19. I love God because He first loved me! I made it personal. Who wouldn't wanna spend time with someone who has made such attempts to show unconditional love and acceptance without having to *do* anything worthy of it! If a man on earth did grand gestures of love, you would at least talk to him, right?

So then how do we pray? Well let's start with how not to pray. The answer to that is found in Matthew 6:5 when Jesus is teaching. He says, "When you pray, don't be like the hypocrites who love to pray publicly on the streets and corners and in the synagogues where everyone can see them. I tell you the truth, that is all the reward they will ever get. But when you pray, go away by yourself, shut the door

SPIRITUAL WELLNESS

behind you, and pray to your Father in private. Then your Father, who sees everything, will reward you. When you pray, don't babble on and on as the Gentiles do. They think their prayers are answered merely by repeating their words again and again. Don't be like them, for your Father knows exactly what you need even before you ask him!" So we know that prayer is a personal communication between us and our Father. It is not superficial. It is not a long and wordy monologue for the purpose of showing other people.

Jesus also tells us something about prayer in Luke 18:10–12 in this parable:

Two men went to the temple to pray. One was a Pharisee and the other was a despised tax collector. The Pharisee stood by himself and prayed this prayer. I thank you, God, that I am not like the other people- cheaters, sinners, adulterers. I'm certainly not like that tax collector! I fast twice a week and I give you a tenth of my income.

Verse 14 summarizes the parable by saying this about prayer, "For all those who exalt themselves will be humbled and those who humble themselves will be exalted." So now we know that prayer does not exalt ourselves while putting down another person. Prayer has everything to do with the heart. You need a heart that is humbled.

James 4:2–3 says that you don't have what you want because you don't ask God for it. And even when you ask, you don't get it because your motives are all wrong—you only want what will give you pleasure.

So now we know that prayer requires having the proper motive. The inner motive must line up with who God is and is not purely self-seeking.

Jesus was asked again about how to pray, and He revealed the "Our Father" prayer to them. He then went on to another parable, highlighting another element of prayer. In Luke 11:5–8, He says the following:

Suppose you went to a friend's house at midnight, wanting to borrow three loaves of bread. You say to him, "A friend of mine has just arrived for a visit, and I have nothing for him to eat." And suppose he calls out from the bedroom, "Don't bother me. The door is locked for the night, and my family and I are all in bed. I can't help you." But I tell you this—though he won't do it for friendship's sake, if you keep knocking long enough, he will get up and give you whatever you need because of your shameless persistence.

Jesus encourages them that in prayer, be persistent. He says to them to keep on asking, keep on seeking, and keep on knocking! He guarantees that everyone who asks will receive. Everyone who seeks will find. Everyone who knocks will have the door opened to them. Prayer is persistent.

In prayers of supplication, no one can tell you word for word what to say to God because everybody's needs are different. Everyone's personality is different. I would also venture to say that everybody's communication with God is different. I explain my situation to God very plainly. I express my feeling plainly. I even confess things out of my heart plainly.

My conversations with God are respectful, but my delivery is as though I'm talking to my earthly father. The important things to remember are to be personable, be real, be humbled, and be persistent in prayer!

SECTION 2.

SPIRITUAL WELLNESS

Spiritual Wellness Step Check

Congratulations! You finished chapter 2! I made this simplified step checklist to summarize what we have learned. I suggest keeping a picture of it in your phone's photo album. This stuff requires practice until it becomes second nature.

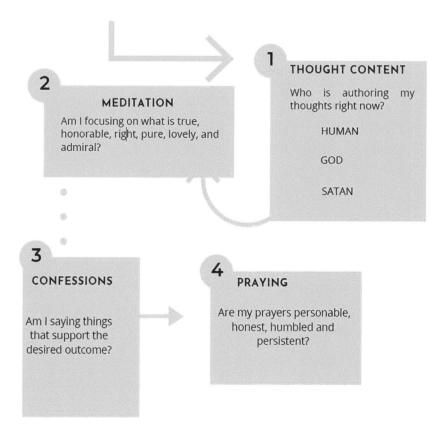

2 MEDITATION
Am I focusing on what is true, honorable, right, pure, lovely, and admiral?

1 THOUGHT CONTENT
Who is authoring my thoughts right now?

HUMAN

GOD

SATAN

3 CONFESSIONS
Am I saying things that support the desired outcome?

4 PRAYING
Are my prayers personable, honest, humbled and persistent?

NOTES

NOTES

NOTES

_____
_____
_____
_____
_____
_____
_____
_____
_____
_____
_____
_____
_____
_____
_____
_____
_____
_____
_____
_____
_____
_____
_____
_____
_____

Section 3.

PHYSICAL WELLNESS

HAND CARE

One of the costs of working in the field of cosmetology is the wear and tear of the body. I'm not just talking about the fatigue at the end of the workday. I'm also talking about the long-term effects on our bodies over time.

When we attend beauty school, they make every mention of proper footwear, the importance of diet and exercise, hand positions when cutting hair, and proper body posture. Due to the bliss of my youthfulness, most of that information got tossed out the window right after graduation. It didn't seem like much more than a bunch of boring statistical data. Needless to say, I got hit with my first bout of bodily breakdown pretty early on. I then become more compliant with the physical wellness precautions of my industry.

I became licensed in cosmetology in 2007. I went right into the hair industry and started servicing clients with my full range of cosmetology service menu. I would do a full head of foil highlights, followed by a pedicure, followed by a sew-in, and then a facial. I did that for about three years before I said to myself that it is time to pick a lane. The mere notion of me continuing to run all over the road of cosmetology made my body ache!

I almost chose the skin and nail avenue, but finally, I decided to focus on haircutting and hair coloring. Since I didn't put into practice all that I learned about hand and body health, it didn't take long for things to begin to rip at the seams.

By 2010, I wore my hands down so badly with my lack of care

that I was starting to experience numbness in my hands while servicing guests. Some might call that a feeling of a limb going to *sleep*. That went on for weeks, and then it started to happen very frequently. I didn't stop working hard nor did I seek medical professional assistance at this point. The happenings began to intensify with very painful pins and needles sensations that would wake me up out of my sleep. It was at that point that I decided it was time to talk to someone about what's happening with my hands.

I googled my symptoms, and a condition called carpal tunnel syndrome came up as the source. I made an appointment for a consultation with a specialist that week.

I met with the specialist. He had me fill out a questionnaire, and he examined my hands. After a series of tests, he determined that I was a candidate for corrective surgery. He laid out a description of what that would entail. It would require for him to slice across the palms of both my hands to relieve the pressure exerted on the median nerve

within the carpal tunnel. The healing time alone would have been six weeks! I was *not* down for that. Instead, I seriously got down before God and asked Him to intervene on my behalf. I couldn't deal with the pain, and I wouldn't do the surgery.

Shortly after that, I was volunteering at the Texas International Hair show, and I met the man who would be my mentor. In one of his haircutting classes, he spent some time talking about carpal tunnel syndrome, treatment, and mostly prevention. I felt like he was talking directly to me.

I absorbed everything he said and quickly put those things into practice. Not only did that divine-ordered knowledge make its way to me, but it also worked for me! It took some time for the effects to be reversed, but I no longer struggle with that painful condition, and I had no hand surgery either.

If you don't currently use any sort of hand-strengthening techniques, then I have some very simple ones to share with you. I call it the haircutter's workout.

PHYSICAL WELLNESS

Who should be doing the haircutter's workout?

- If your tools of the trade include clippers, razors, or shears
- If you work with tint brushes daily
- If you do offer hair-sewing services

What is Carpel Tunnel Syndrome?

Pain, tingling, and numbness in your hands due to excess pressure in your wrist and on the median nerve. Usually caused by repetitive tasks

SECTION 3.

PHYSICAL WELLNESS

The following chart maps out the different types of wrist and hand stretches you can incorporate into your daily habits. Do each of them for three to five minutes a day, preferably just before a hair service requiring a repetitive wrist movement.

Hand stretching

Slowly take one hand and push back the palm of the other hand until the fingers are bend toward the forearm. Then reverse the stretch until the fingers bend toward the inner arm.

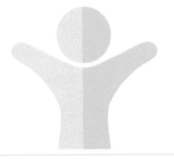

Air piano

With your hands straight out, imitate the fingers playing piano. Move your fingers as far as rapidly as you can using the full range of motion your fingers will allow.

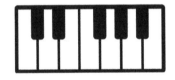

Wrist circles

First, bend both your wrists forward then create full circling motions clockwise. Then create full wrist circles counterclockwise.

Wrist flapping

Bend your hand at the wrist and leave them limp. Now using the weight of the arm and leaving the wrist limp, allow the hands to flap back and forth.

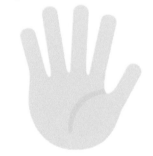

PHYSICAL WELLNESS

BACK CARE

We just went over some information to keep our hands healthy, so now let's discuss our bodies. I want to start by telling you about how my back was affected by my being so passionate about customer service. Let me explain.

Remember I told you earlier that when I first graduated from beauty school, I did everything my license allowed. Then I specialized in cut and color. While doing cuts and color jobs, my clients would get so relaxed by my touch. They would be so relaxed that they would either close their eyes or nod off into a little nap. I would feel so complimented by the trust that they had in me. It was the fact that first-time guests wouldn't feel the need to watch me! The other side of that coin is that a sleeping client could not adjust as I needed access to certain parts of the head and neck.

Allowing that sort of deep relaxation in the chair meant working my back in ways that I should not have done. I would twist and contort my body to cut hair in ways that would have me injured by the end of the day. It's already a toll on the body when coloring and cutting all day. I didn't need to add more to that situation. That went on for some time before I said I have to do something different.

I wanted to keep the relaxing element of my service but not get hurt in the process. I learned to separate it. I gave extended scalp massage and installed a back massager under hair dryers. The new deal required that the client stay awake in the chair and work with me.

PHYSICAL WELLNESS

Back pain can be a natural side effect of hairdressing. I experienced bodily discomfort within the first five years of my career, not because I wasn't practicing proper posture or any of the other proper practices either. We will get to that soon.

The most common complaints are pain and pressure in between the shoulder blades and upper back. This is said to be due to the continuous standing for extended periods of time coupled with the posture practiced by the cosmetologist.

In case you forgot what the proper posture is for our line of work, I'll remind you. Take the footing stance with your feet shoulder-width apart. That means to have your feet positioned in line with the outer frame of your shoulders.

Also make sure that while you're working, your arms are not higher than the height of your shoulders. Working with the arms raised higher than that will exhaust the muscles a lot quicker. Envision your elbows positioned on an invisible dinner table.

In addition to the position in which we stand, we have tools in the salon to keep us from damaging our posture. We just have to remember to use them according to their purpose.

HYDRAULIC CHAIR

The general purpose of the hydraulic salon chair is to elim-inate the need for the stylist to stoop, bend, and contort while servicing clients. Yet we still find ourselves doing the most when it comes to fine detail work. I've seen some stylists over the years use their chair correctly until it comes the time to fine-tune, and then the detachment from their regimented ways occur.

Remember I told you about my clients being lulled to sleep while getting serviced? I was just using my chair as a place to seat my client, and that was all! Can you just imagine what I was putting my back through while trying to service a drooping head?

We have to remember to keep our posture and use the chair as a tool and not just fine furniture. If you find yourself feeling the need to stoop, then stop the service and adjust the chair to the higher height needed to reach. I know that seems like a pain to keep raising and lowering the chair. Consider this. Your client is getting her hair done one time in the course of that day. You may be just bending one or two times to cut, press, or reach that hard-to-reach section. Multiply that cut corner practice across all the clients you serve in a week. That compound interest is not in your favor. Believe me, it is better to retrain yourself and save your back.

PROFESSIONAL TOOLS

Another thing worthy of discussing is the importance of the thermal tools we need for bodily longevity. I remember when we got our tool kits in beauty school. That kit had every tool we would need to start our hair journey. It was valued at a little over a thousand dollars back then! But what I came to understand was that professional tools would save me time and effort over the course of my career. I never ascribed to the "just get the cheapest tool" frame of thought. Once I had a taste of what a difference quality-made tools could do for me, I was completely convinced.

Let's say for instance having a professional blow dryer versus a household one.

Pro dryers are usually lighter, fast-drying, and have healthier heating elements. These will all come in handy for a stylist who has five to ten blowouts in a day.

Having the capacity to spend fewer minutes per guest and handing lighter-weight tools with less effort to smooth the hair are all good news for the hands and back. That's actually lowering the risk for repetitive strain injury.

Investing in tools is expensive, but the benefits outweigh the cost in the end. In addition to the bodily benefits, good pro-tools will actually yield more polished results than low-quality tools.

HAIRSTYLIST DIET

It has been said that Americans have an upside-down relationship with food. We live to eat and not eat to live! We are emotional eaters, addictive eaters, and even celebratory eaters. Not enough of us are purely nutritional eaters.

In the beauty industry, we have a running joke about something called the hairstylists' diet. It is when a beauty professional eats nothing for breakfast, works an eight-to-ten-hour shift, and then inhales a one-thousand-two-hundred-calorie meal followed by crashing for the night. It is hilarious because we can all relate! It can be argued that the relationship between beauty professionals and nutrition is also upside-down.

I have been on every end of the spectrum as it relates to nutrition and working.

I was a vegan for three years, pregnant and meal prepping, a fast-food junkie, and even a restaurant lunch break stylist. Each of those lifestyles yielded different results in how my body responded to working long hours.

I wonder how many of us have returned to the salon with our COVID lockdown food tendencies? I will be the first to admit that I have heavier snack habits and less physical endurance behind the chair due to my salon inactivity. Now is the time to set the record straight and put in place some healthier food protocols. After all, our bodies are our temples and the only vehicle we have for our future.

Did you know the human body is worth forty-five million dollars? You are a valuable asset!

MEAL PREPPING

In my experience, the best way to be successful in consuming the fuel we need for the workday is to provide it ourselves. That is called meal prep. Meal prepping involves planning and preparing our food in advance of the time we need to eat it. Like I said before, most of us eat whatever is near the salon. Those items don't typically serve us well. Anything prepared fast is usually fried, and that means sodium. Too much salt can cause the body to retain excess water. That could be a reason one would experience ankle swelling after a workday in the salon.

So how do you know what to pack? One general tip I suggest is to listen to your body. Do you feel aching in your joints? Do you lack energy? Do you get headaches often?

SECTION 3.

PHYSICAL WELLNESS

These are all signs of your body telling you what it needs. So based on your symptoms, choose foods that counter those areas of concern.

Here is a list of common ailments and a few food suggestions to solve them:

  Joint pain: fish oils and ginger root
  Low energy: bananas, salmon, and apples
  Backache: cherry juice and green tea
  Brain frog: avocado and leafy greens
  Bad mood: dark chocolate and berries
  Dehydration: lettuce and cucumber

WATER CONSUMPTION

A lot of people also have a weird relationship with water. As a matter of fact, 80 percent of working Americans say they hate drinking water. That is according to prnewswire.org.

In my personal experience in the salon environment, that totally figures. We like coffee,

energy drinks, juices, and sodas. Not water! But the strange thing is that water is a very essential element we need to combat our ailments.

My goal in this chapter is to help you understand the importance of water. I hope that we can look at water as a life source and not a bland-tasting beverage. After all, our bodies are made up of 60 percent of the stuff!

For example, some general headaches come from dehydration and can be solved by drinking water and restoring electrolytes.

I know plenty of ladies who complain about bloating, and that can be solved and prevented by drinking the right amount of water. There's also a whole science about people mistaking thirst for hunger because of the weakness of the thirst signals in the brain.

I often get asked the age-old question, "What can I put on my hair to make it grow?" I always start with what you put in your body. Water. Dehydration immediately stunts hair growth! Not to mention, it puts us at higher risk for viral, bacterial, and urinary tract infections!

Recommended H_2O intake: men: 101 ounces; women: 74 ounces

VITAMIN SUPPLEMENTS

The topic of vitamins is very controversial. People are either all for it or not interested at all.

I used to represent the side that was not at all interested, but I began to notice minor health declines by my late twenties. That caused me to look at my regimens more closely. Not to mention by this time in life, my husband had become what I affectionately declared "King Vitamin!" We ate virtually the same things, but there was an edge that he had with energy, vitality, and even mood! That was largely because he took vitamins and supplements for what his body was lacking in production. I'm in no way suggesting that blindly purchasing a bunch of vitamins from GNC is the answer to all health issues.

I'm urging that seeking a medical professional and testing to see what, if any, vitamin deficiency is there and adding that to the body.

As we speak, Texas has lifted the COVID restrictions. Salons will begin to reopen at full capacity, and mingling with people will soon begin. There are two suggestions I would like to share.

Going back into social situations, it's recommended that we not be deficient in vitamin C. Vitamin C is responsible for boosting the immune system. That will come in handy when encountering the general public.

According to a Harvard study, vitamin D is recommended for all of us for COVID protection. It's not a cure, but it will certainly help to build a wall of defense. Vitamin D is important because it is responsible for our body's defense against viruses and bacteria. We may be deficient in this particular nutrient because of the prolonged periods of lockdown and work-from-home culture. We normally produce this nutrient from exposure to the sun.

NOTES

NOTES

NOTES

ABOUT THE AUTHOR

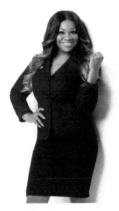

Robin "Honey" George is a University of Louisiana at Lafayette 2005 bachelor of science graduate turned licensed cosmetologist in 2006. In 2013, she started her own brand of educational and inspirational hair training sessions called the Honey George experience.

Her unique spin on traditional cosmetology training combined with her warm personality, systematic techniques, and inspirational concepts keeps her students heavily engaged.

In her career, she has taught on many platforms nationwide including Chews Multicultural Hair Affair, Bronner Brothers, the Extensions Expo, and the Beauty Conn, to name a few.

After overcoming her own mental battles brought on by the devastation of COVID-19, she now aims to share her journey and assist beauty industry professionals to obtain their mental and spiritual wellness.

As a man thinketh in his heart, so is he
—Proverbs 23:7